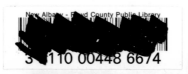

Dance

Barry Gibson

Heinemann Library
Chicago, Illinois

Customer Service 888-454-2279

Designed by Ken Vail Graphic Design
Illustrations by Graham-Cameron Illustration (Sarah Hedley)
Printed by Wing King Tong in Hong Kong

04 03 02 01 00
10 9 8 7 6 5 4 3 2 1

Library of Congress Cataloging in Publication Data
Gibson, Barry.
    Dance / Barry Gibson.
        p. cm. – (You can do it!)
    Summary: An introduction to dance, describing styles and steps, with tips on safety, warmups, and cooldowns.
    Includes bibliographical references (p.) and index.
    ISBN 1-57572-960-1 (library bdg.)
    1. Dance Juvenile literature. [1. Dance.] I. Title.
II. Series: You can do it! (Des Plaines, Ill.)
GV1596.5.G53 1999
792.8—dc21   99-22660
                         CIP

Acknowledgments
The publishers would like to thank Jaqui Isow and the students of Bishops Stortford School of Performing Arts for all their help in the preparation of this book.

The publishers would like to thank the following for permission to reproduce photographs: Trevor Clifford, pages 4, 5, 6, 8, 10, 19, 22; Dee Conway, pages 14, 16, 17 (top and bottom), 20 (bottom); Corbis, page 12; Performing Arts, page 20 (top).

Cover photograph reproduced with permission of Collections/Anthea Sieveking.

Every effort has been made to contact copyright holders of any material reproduced in this book. Any omissions will be rectified in subsequent printings if notice is given to the publisher.

Some words are shown in bold, **like this.** You can find out what they mean by looking in the Glossary.

Contents

Dance and You

To dance, your body needs to be able to move.

Wear light, comfortable clothes so you can move easily.

shoulder

arm

bottom

leg

head

hand

foot

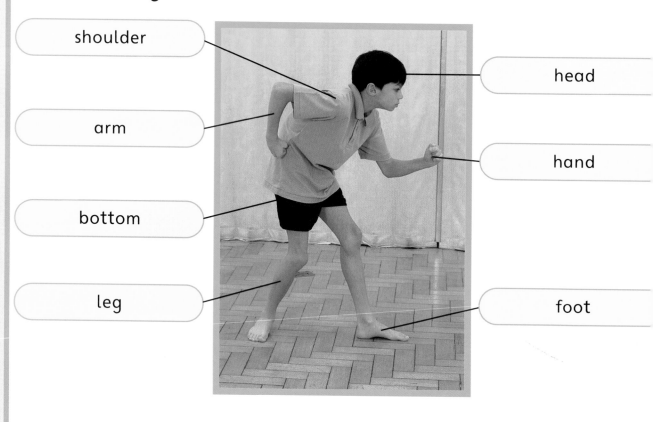

You will need some music, too.

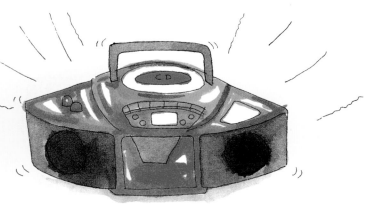

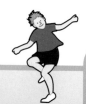

Begin by walking in different ways. Try walking strong and heavy. Then walk gentle and light.

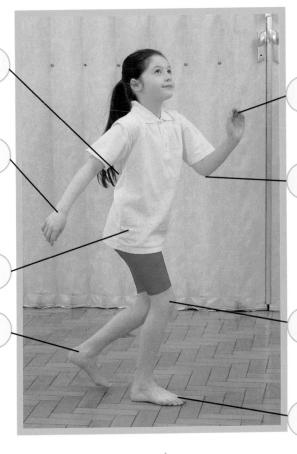

back

fingers

wrist

elbow

hip

ankle

knee

toes

SAFETY STAR

Usually bare feet are best. Make sure the floor is clean and not rough.

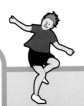

Are You Ready?

Before you dance, make sure your body is ready. This is called a **warm-up**. You need to warm up all the different parts of your body, especially your muscles.

Start by bending, swinging, or **stretching**.

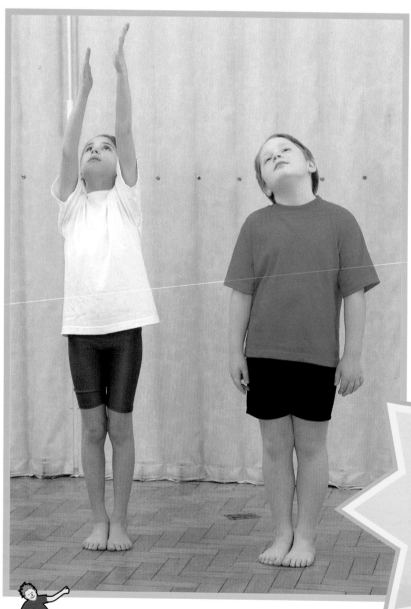

SAFETY STAR

Always warm up your body before you dance so that you don't hurt yourself.

Try these movements to warm up your whole body!

Touch your toes.

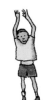
Stretch up high.

Wiggle your fingers.

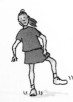
Wiggle your toes.

Wiggle your elbows.

Wiggle your nose.

Shake your shoulders.

Roll your head.

Swing from side to side.

Turn around.

Walk in place.

Run in place.

Breathe deep and rest. Now, let's dance!

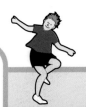

Let's Move!

Here are some ways to move your feet.

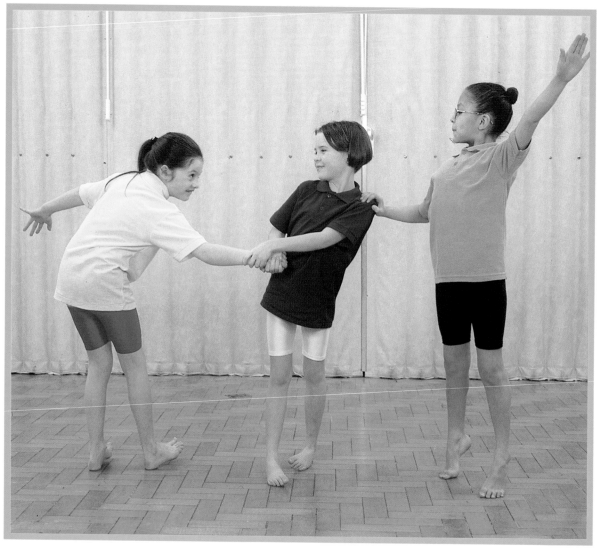

Step with your heels.

Step with the sides of your feet.

Step only on your tiptoes.

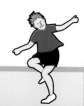

Your body can leap, hop, skip, and jump. You can move like animals do.

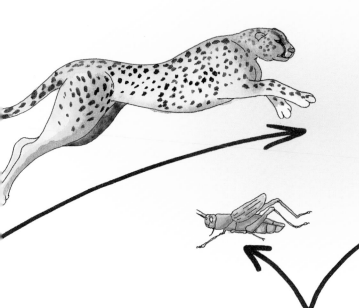

There are many ways to turn and twist your body.

Try to spin and twist.

SAFETY STAR

Never land on your knees. Be careful not to fall.

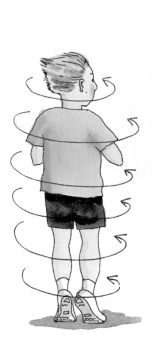
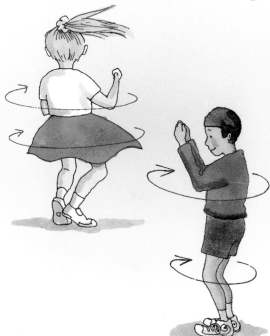
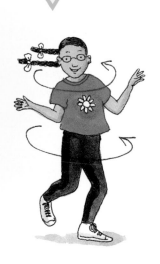

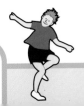

Which Way Shall We Go?

You can move yourself in different directions.

Try going forward, backward, and sideways.

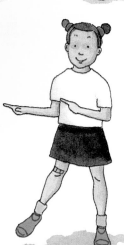

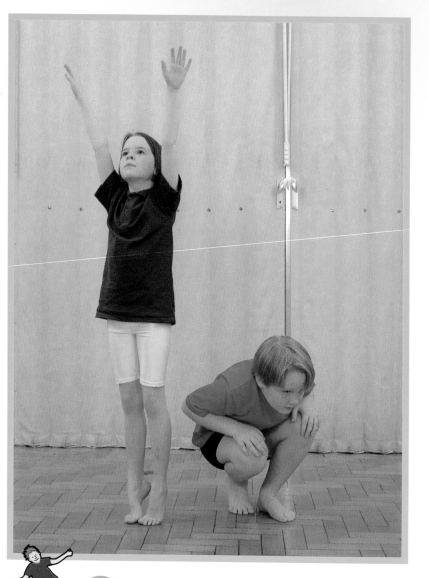

These children are rising high in the air and sinking low to the ground.

Imagine you are looking down from the ceiling. See the footstep patterns on the floor? Try to follow them.

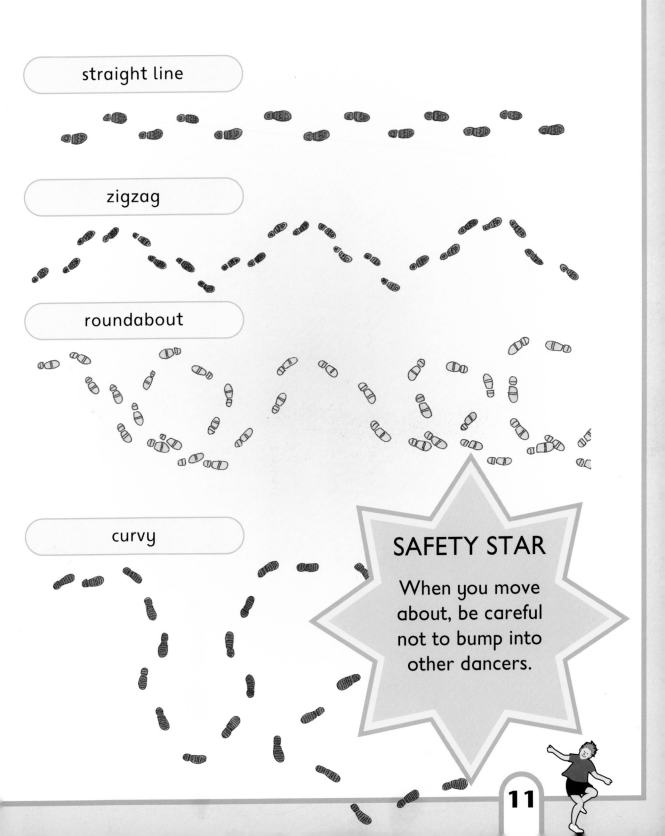

straight line

zigzag

roundabout

curvy

SAFETY STAR

When you move about, be careful not to bump into other dancers.

Move Together

In a dance space, a group of people can make all kinds of shapes. They can make lines, rows, squares, and circles.

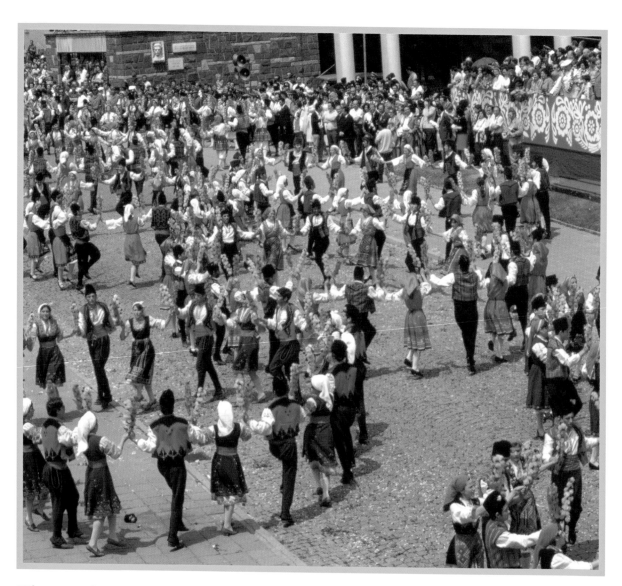

These dancers are doing a huge circle dance from Bulgaria. It is being performed at the Festival of Roses.

It is also fun to work with a partner.

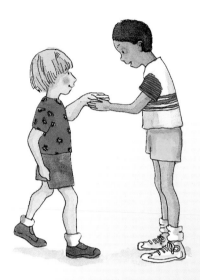 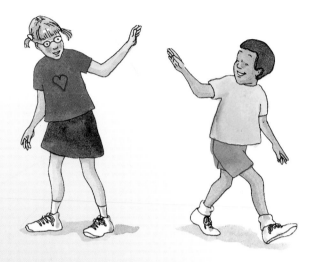

You can meet . . .   and you can part.

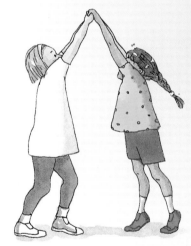 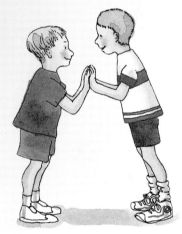

You can make an
arch together.

You can gently push and
pull each other without
falling over.

SAFETY STAR

Help your partner
balance safely.
Support them
well.

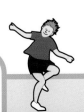

Step in Time

Dance and music go together well.

Some dances are fast.

Here is a Kathak dancer from India.

Her feet are tapping the floor very quickly.

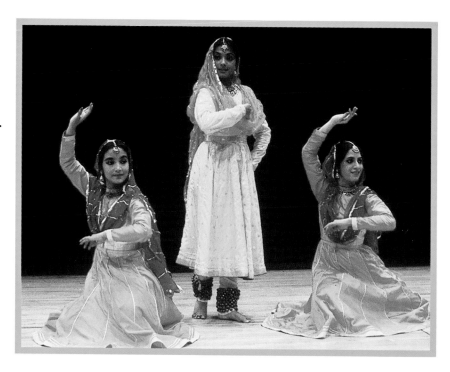

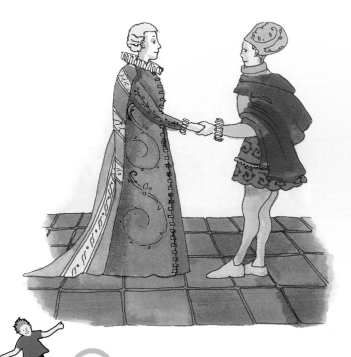

Some dances are slow and steady.

This dance is called a Pavane. It was first danced about 400 years ago.

People thought the smooth, proud movements were like a peacock's.

Rhythm is the way music and sounds make patterns in time. In dance music, rhythm helps you know when to move.

Sometimes, music has a strong **beat**.

Here are some moves to do in time to music.

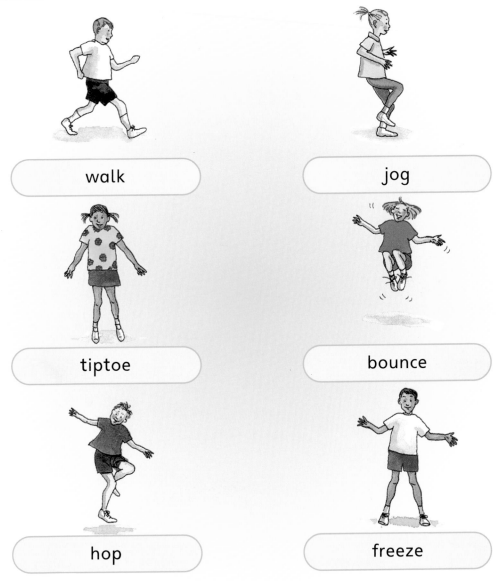

walk

jog

tiptoe

bounce

hop

freeze

Feel the rhythm in your feet!

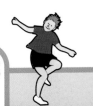

What's the Idea?

Dance is also a way of sharing ideas with an **audience**. A dance can create a **mood**. It may make the audience feel happy or sad. It may even tell a story.

Dances from a certain time or place are often done in a special **style**.

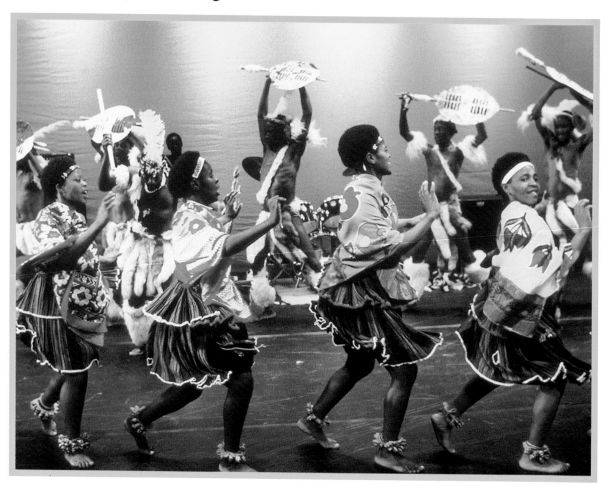

How would you describe the style of this dance?

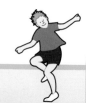

Each style of dance needs a different kind of dance **energy**. Sometimes a style has special steps.

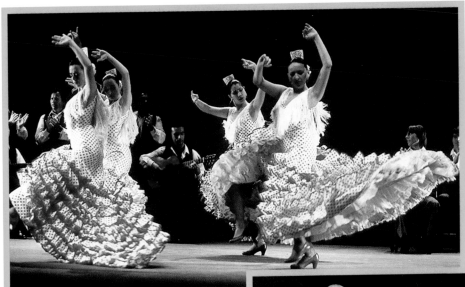

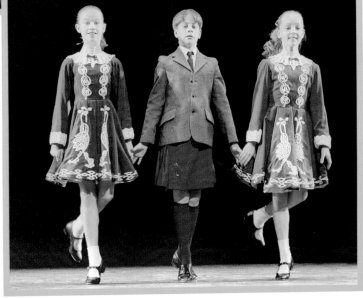

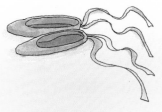

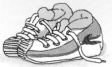

For some kinds of dance, the dancers wear special shoes.

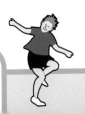

Who Am I?

Have you ever wanted to pretend to be someone or something else?

By moving in special ways, you can be a different **character** in an instant!

Pretend to be these characters. What movements and **gestures** will you make?

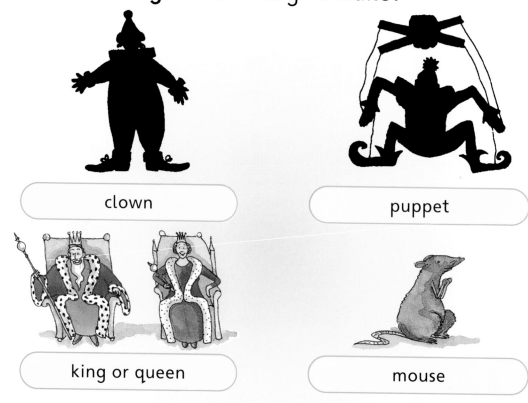

clown

puppet

king or queen

mouse

Your dance can show the characters as they change their **moods**. Are the characters scared? Happy? Sad? Angry?

Put your dance ideas together to tell a story.

These children are pretending to be a machine.

Each person makes a different movement.

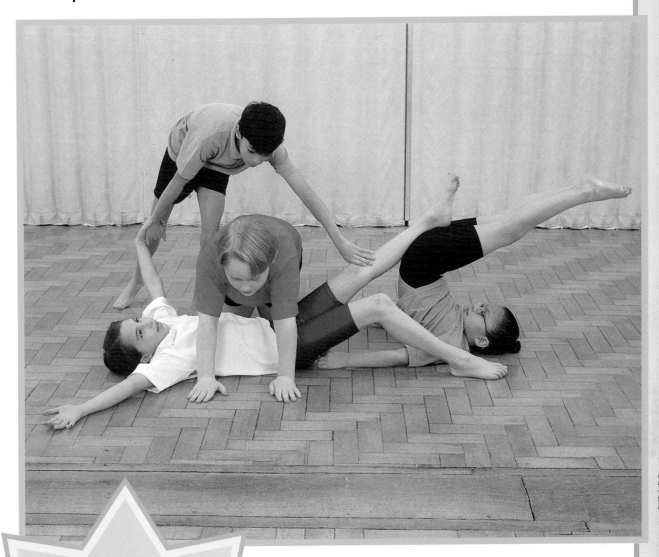

SAFETY STAR

In a group dance, avoid bumps and falls. Lean against and hold each other carefully!

Keep Your Eyes Open!

Dancers sometimes wear special costumes.

They might also use special **props**. Props are objects, such as chairs or books, that are used in the **performance**.

How would you use a prop in your dance?

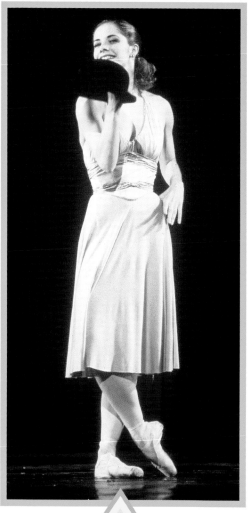

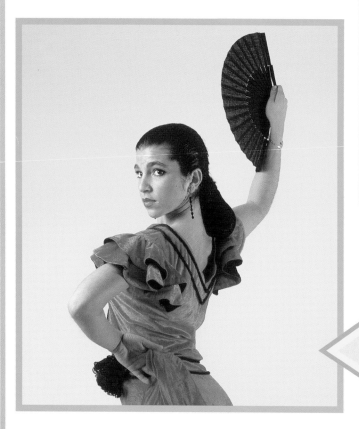

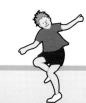

SAFETY STAR

Check the props to be sure that they are safe to use.

Every dance that tells a story needs a beginning, a middle, and an end.

Movements put together can make a **sequence**.

Some dance **styles** have special sequences called **routines**.

The steps are very lively in a rock'n'roll routine.

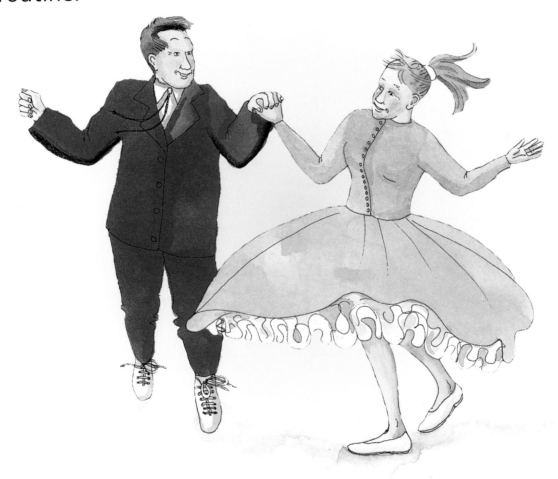

A **choreographer** is the person who decides which moves go into a dance.

Be a choreographer. Plan a routine of movements for a group of dancers.

Cool It!

After using lots of **energy**, you need to let your body calm down.

After all that work, you might feel tired.

Your arms and legs might ache a little.

You might feel hot. So, cool it!

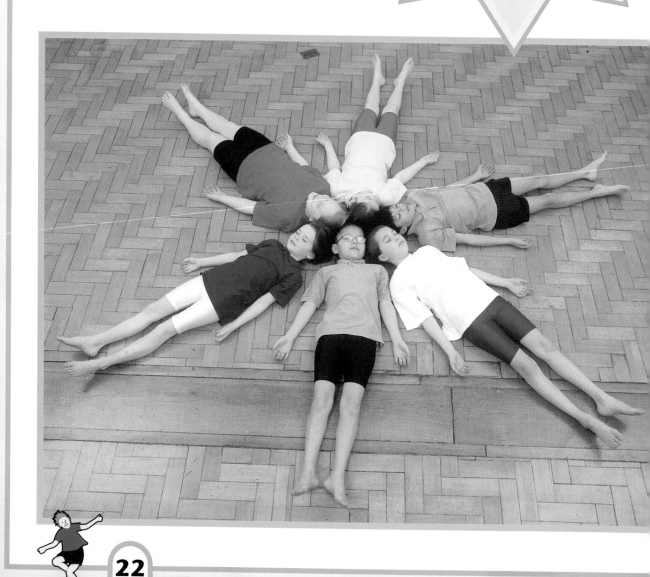

22

Here is a step-by-step way to cool down.

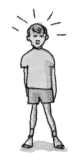

1. Stand still and close your eyes.

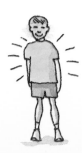

2. Breathe with slow, deep breaths.

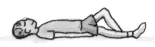

3. Now lie on your back.

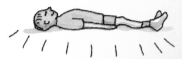

4. Let your body sink into the floor.

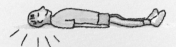

5. Relax your head. Let it go loose.

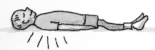

6. Relax your shoulders.

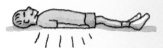

7. Relax your arms.

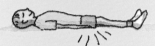

8. Relax your fingers.

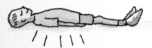

9. Relax your back.

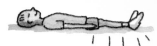

10 Relax your legs.

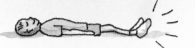

11 Relax your toes.

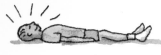

12 Slowly open your eyes.

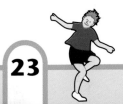

Glossary

audience group of people watching a performance

beat repeating sound that marks the rhythm in music

character person or creature

choreographer person who chooses the movements of a dance

cool-down way of moving to relax after exercise

energy power that helps you to move

gestures body movements that express an idea

mood how people are feeling

performance event in which you dance for an audience

prop object used in a show, such as a table or chair

routine set of dance steps

rhythm regular pattern of sounds

sequence way that movements follow one another

stretching moving muscles at the joints as far as possible

style special way of dancing

warm-up exercises that get the body ready to dance

Index

More Books to Read

Ancona, George. *Let's Dance.* New York: William Morrow & Company, 1998.

Bailey, Donna. *Dancing.* Austin, Tex.: Raintree Steck-Vaughn, 1991.

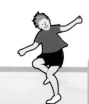